Thank You for purchasing this Quick Knowledge e-book

I0435474

Copyright © 2016 Mano Hano
All rights reserved worldwide. No part of this publication may be replicated, redistributed, or given away in any form without the prior written consent of the author.
Contact information: manal120@yahoo.com

Limit of Liability/Disclaimer of Warranty
Nothing on this eBooks is intended to provide medical advice, diagnosis or treatment. Although every precaution has been taken to verify the accuracy of the information contained herein, the publisher assumes no responsibility for any errors or omissions. No liability is assumed for damages that may result from the use of information contained within.

Contents

Banned By other Countries but is a main staple of our diet!

Introduction

Genetically engineered foods are foods which have had foreign genes from other plants inserted into their genetic codes. The Food and Drug Administration (FDA) approves and regulates the use of genetically modified organisms (GMO's), which are foods treated to be more resistant to disease, to enhance their nutritional value and so they are able to grow in harsher climates.

However, the genetic modification of crops happens so frequently, that in the U.S. it is nearly impossible to find natural organic versions. This is mainly down to farmers crop dusting their seeds so they become genetically resistant to specific weed-killers, or to repel bugs from plants.

As a result, many of the foods we eat will contain ingredients derived from GMO's. And with no indication as to if the food you are eating has been tampered with, it means you should be considerate and understand what you are consuming on a daily basis. It is easier to avoid GM foods in Europe thanks to laws which require statuary labelling on all packaging. There is no such law in the U.S.

or Canada. This is why we find ourselves in a situation where some foods are banned in Europe due to health risks, yet readily available in the U.S. and Canada.

You should keep an eye out for the following banned foods.

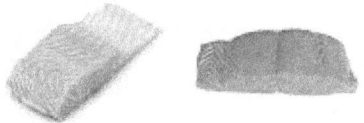

Spot the Difference: Stripes of Fat are visible on Farmed Salmon. No stripes of Fat are visible on Wild Salmon.

What is Farm-Raised Salmon?

Salmon aquaculture (farming) is the industrial production of salmon from egg to market in a net-cage, pond or contained system. Farmed salmon is larger in scale and contains higher amounts of Omega-3s.

Why it's not good for you?

Salmon raised in captivity are fed on grains mixed with antibiotics and other prescription drugs. This diet results in developing an unappetising gray colour, and to compensate they are fed a synthetic astaxanthin made out of petrochemicals, something not approved for human consumption. Salmon raised on these substances contain much more potentially harmful contaminants than wild salmon, and are banned in Australia and in New Zealand. (Natural, 2013)

What is the Alternative?

Wild salmon is much more expensive and is commonly prized for its health benefits. It is a fatty fish that is loaded with Omega-3 fatty acids, which is a healthy addition to any diet. However, the price and access to wild salmon is often a reason why people opt for farmed salmon.

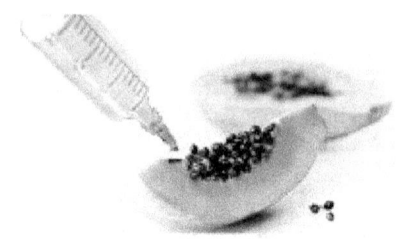

What is Genetically Engineered Papaya?

Papayas are one of the most common genetically modified (GMO) crops in America, mainly thanks to an outbreak of a papaya ring virus which allowed scientists to genetically modify it. These new modified papaya plants are no longer susceptible to infection, allowing farmers to cultivate the fruit even when the virus is widespread.

Why it's not Good for you?

Most Hawaiian papaya is now genetically engineered to be resistant to the ringspot virus. Mounting research now shows that animals which eat genetically engineered foods suffer a wide range of maladies, including intestinal damage, multiple-organ damage, massive tumours, birth defects, premature death, and near complete sterility by the third generation of offspring. Genetically engineered papaya is banned in the EU. (McClees, 2015)

What is the Alternative?

Papayas are rich in Vitamins A and C, thus considered one of the healthiest foods available. It is loaded with the enzyme papain, which helps you digest protein.

Most papayas from Mexico and from Belize are not genetically modified. Look for the following: The Mexican Red (red flesh), Kapoho, Caribbean Red, Maradol, Singapore Pink (bright orange flesh), and the Higgins variety (a bright yellow flesh) are healthy natural papayas. (McClees, 2015).

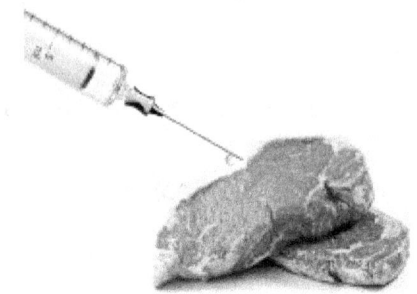

What is Tainted Meat?

Tainted meat occurs when a drug is fed to the cattle in the final weeks before slaughter to *"improve the rate at which the animals convert feed to lean muscle"* rather than fat. Since industrial factory-farmed animals are usually excessively fat due to lack of exercise, ractopamine is used to generate more lean meat.

Due to the addition of ractopamine, American beef, pork, and turkeys are now considered sub-standard in more than 100 countries. The U.S government still openly allows its continual use. (Fake, 2013)

Why it's not Good for you?

In both pigs and cattle, ractopamine leads to excessive food cravings, anorexia, bloat, respiratory issues, hoof problems, lameness, tightness, stress and overt aggression.

Ractopamine is also proven to affect the human cardiovascular system, and is considered responsible for hyperactivity along with possible chromosomal abnormalities and behavioural changes. Ractopamine is banned in 160 countries in Europe, Taiwan, Russia and Mainland China. (Natural, 2013)

What is the Alternative?

Other than checking the food labels on all meat for ractopamine, consider purchasing 100% organic, grass fed meat.

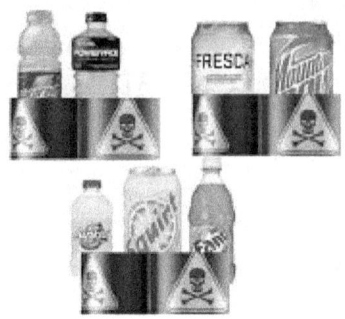

What is Flame Retardant Drink?

Brominated veggie oil is a synthetic chemical substance called BVO. It contains bromine that is used as a flame retardant inside plastics, upholstered household furniture, and some clothing for children.

Why it's not Good for you?

Citrus-flavored soda as well as sports drinks sold in the US typically include BVO, which was originally copyrighted by chemical substance companies like a flame retardant. BVO has shown to be able to bioaccumulate throughout human tissue and breasts milk, and animal studies have discovered it causes reproductive as well as behavioral troubles in large doses. (DrWeil, 2013)

Coca-Cola's recently removed BVO from its Powerade drinks is evidence that food makers are coming under pressure for the ingredients they use in their products. BVO is not approved for food utilities in Japan and Europe.

What is the Alternative?

Filtered water, iced tea, and sparkling water mixed with a little natural fruit juice.

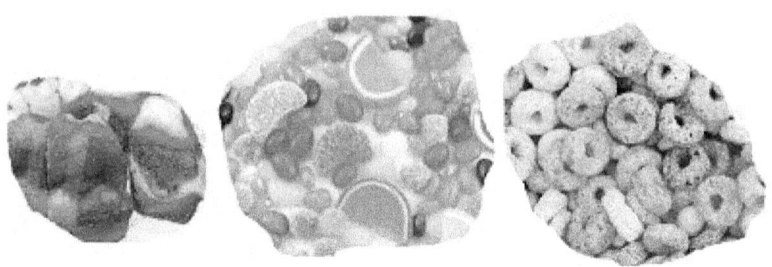

What is Processed Food?

The phrase 'processed food' leans to describe any food that has been altered from their natural state. These foods have been processed extensively in order to be edible, and include chemicals to alter food coloring to maintain or help the appearance of the food. Processed food are often packaged in boxes, cans or bags.

Why it's not Good for you?

In excess of 3,000 food preservatives - flavorings, colors and other ingredients - are added to US foods despite studies which show toxicity and dangerous health effects, especially regarding adverse effects on kids behavior. It is these side effects which lead to a European law in 2010 which required warning labels on foods that contain certain artificial colors. (Natural, 2013)

In the UK, Kraft, Coca-Cola, and Mars were forced to remove artificial colors, sodium benzoate, and aspartame from their product lines as a result of consumer pressure and government recommendations.

What is the Alternative?

The more whole, nutritious, unprocessed foods you eat, the less likely you are to run into artificial dyes. Always check food labels, and avoid anything with terms such as "FD&C Lakes" (a type of dye pigment), "Citrus Crimson, " or "artificial color. " Some stores have done the job for you: Most natural markets, including co-ops, Whole Foods Markets, and Trader Joe's, exclusively use natural dyes in their processed foods.

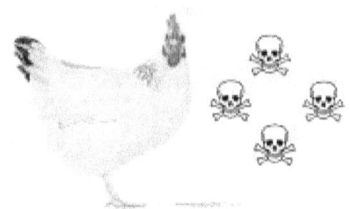

What is Arsenic-Laced Chicken

Chicken feed is laced with a drug in order to speed up its growth, improve meat pigmentation and prevent disease. Arsenic-based drugs are approved for used in animal feed in the US because they create animals grow more rapidly and make this meat appear pinker (i. age. "fresher").

Why it's not good for you?

Arsenical chemicals like roxarsone have been in use since the 1940s and as we now know, these chemicals are pervasive, and are known to cause harm. (Huff, 2013) The FDA claims they are safe simply because they contain organic arsenic, which is less toxic as opposed to other inorganic type, which is the known carcinogen. Nonetheless, studies suggest this organic arsenic can easily transform into inorganic arsenic.

It's well-established that carcinogens are linked with increased risk levels in various types of cancers, cause endocrine and defence mechanisms dysfunctions in addition to a range of cognitive disorders (such as learning disabilities, memory difficulties and poor concentration). (U.S. 2015)

After a study by the FDA, it was agreed to withdraw just three of the four arsenicals on the market: roxarsone, carbarsone, and arsanilic acid. The fourth drug, nitarsone, is still allowed in the feed supply . This drug is another feed additive known to increase growth, weight, and prevent avian disease and is made by the same companies that made other arsenicals (Ly,2013)

The European Union, Japan and many other countries determined the drugs as unsafe and does not permit arsenic-based drugs in food.

What is the Alternative?

Always go out of your way to find locally raised, free-range organic and natural chicken.

Bread with Potassium Bromate

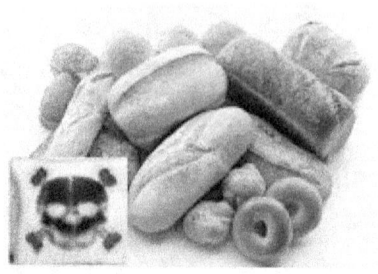

What is Bread with Potassium Bromate?

Potassium Bromate is added to flour to strengthen the dough and allow it to rise higher and add to the finished bread an attractive white color.

Why it's not good for you?

The use of potassium Bromate as an additive to commercial bakery goods is a heavy contributor to bromide overstock in Western cultures. Bromated flour is "enriched" with Potassium Bromate. Scientific research has discovered links with Potassium Bromate to kidney and neuroregeneration damage, thyroidal problems, gastrointestinal pain, and cancer.

It is required in California for all food with potassium bromate to carry a warning label, and the use of potassium bromate is prohibited in Canada, China, Brazil and European Union. (Aguayo, 2015)

What is the Alternative?

Do not purchase foods that have "bromated flour" or "potassium bromate" in their list of ingredients. All other flours are fine.

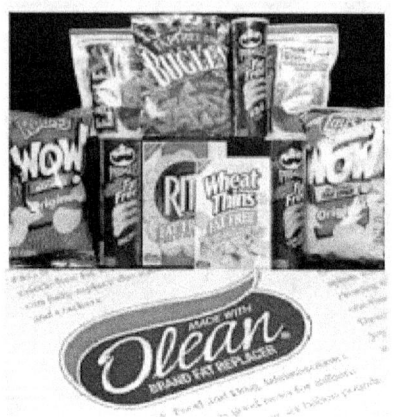

What is Olestra?

Olestra is a fat-free additive found in foods such as fat-free potato chips, french fries and corn chips.

Why it's not good for you?

Olestra, aka Olean, is a calorie and cholesterol-free fat substitute used in fat-free snacks. Adverse reactions include diarrhoea, aches and leaky bowels. Olestra also disturbs the absorption regarding fat soluble vitamins like a, D, E as well as K.

Olestra is banned in England and Canada.

What is the Alternative?

Your very best bet is to stay clear of chips and general processed foods. Rather, eat healthy rich fats found in plants, as well as organic eggs and oils.

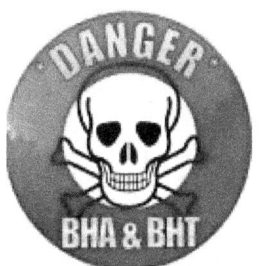

What is Preservatives BHA and BHT?

BHA (butylated hydroxyanisole) and also BHT (butylated hydroxytoluene) are widely used by the foods industry as chemical preservatives to stop oils in ingredients from oxidizing and becoming rancid. Oxidation affects the flavor, coloring and odor involving foods and decreases some nutrients. (Wellness, 2011)

Why it's not good for you?

BHA might cause cancer in rats, and might be a cancer-causing agent in humans too. US experts figured BHA "is reasonably anticipated to be a human carcinogen". BHA, in addition to BHT, are prohibited in Japan and parts of the European Union. The UK does not permit BHA in baby foods.

What is the Alternative?

Limit how many snacks and sweets you eat. A diet of fresh foods which contain very few or no additives are more nutritious overall. You may look for packaged foods that make use of other preservatives, including vitamin E, or don't have any preservatives at all.

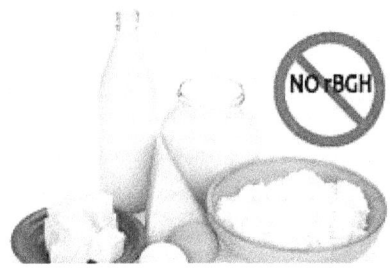

What is Milk and Dairy Products Laced with rBGH?

Recombinant bovine growth hormone (rBGH) is the largest selling dairy animal drug in the US. rBGH is a synthetic version of natural bovine somatotropin (BST), a hormone produced in a cows pituitary glands to boost milk production. Milk, cheese, yogurt and other dairy products are commonly laced with recombinant bovine growth hormone (rBGH).

Why it's not good for you?

rBGH can be a synthetic version of natural bovine somatotropin (BST). It is banned in 30 nations due to its dangers to humans, with health risks to intestines, prostate, as well as encouraging breast cancer by promoting conversion of normal tissue cells into cancerous ones. (Mercola, 2013)

Despite decades of evidence about the dangers of rBGH, the FDA still maintains it's safe for human consumption and ignores all scientific evidence. In 1999, the United Nations Safety Agency ruled unanimously not to endorse or set safety standards for rBGH milk, which has effectively resulted in an international ban on US milk. rBGH is forbidden in Australia, New Zealand, Israel, EU, and Canada

What is the Alternative?

Eating grass-fed meat is the safest option. These foods can be found at local farms and in health food stores. An alternative to rBGH infected dairy products would be to consume raw milk that comes from untreated cows. Look for labeling that says "rBGH-free" or "No rBGH."

Conclusion

Meat—and beef in particular—is a mainstay of the traditional American dinner. Unfortunately, the vast majority of it is filled with harmful additives of one form or another.

Russia is the fourth largest importer of US meats, purchasing about $500 million-worth of beef and pork annually. They issued a ban on US meat imports in February of 2013, and will enforce until the US agrees to certify that all their meat is ractopamine-free. At present, the US does not even test for the presence of this drug in meats sold. (Natural, 2013)

It has been estimated that 70% of all processed foods in the United States contain at least one genetically modified ingredient—usually a product of soy plants. (Genetically, n. d.)

Unlike countries such as Australia and Japan, the United States currently has no laws requiring companies to label products containing genetically modified ingredients. Despite the controversy surrounding them, genetically modified plants have taken root in our world. As with any new technology, members of society have the responsibility to become informed about genetically modified plants, in order to make decisions about their responsible use and regulation.

Other Quick Knowledge Title you might be interested in…….

Quick Knowledge... How to control Anger: The Techniques to defuse your most powerful Emotion.

www.amazon.com/How-Control-Anger-Techniques-Management-ebook/dp/B01C0FCC9E/

Reference

Aguayo. J. (2015) Potassium Bromate. Retrieve from
http://www.ewg.org/research/potassium-bromate

DrWeil. (2013) Q & A library. Retrieve from
http://www.drweil.com/drw/u/QAA401239/Flame-
Retardant-In-Your-Soda.html

Eldred, S. (2014) The truth about Artificial Food coloring.
Retrieve from https://experiencelife.com/article/the-truth-
about-artificial-food-colorings/

Fake Food Watch. (2013). U.S. Pork, Beef laced with Drug
banned in Europe, China, Russia. Retrieve from
http://www.fakefoodwatch.com/2013_02_01_archive.html

Gentic Science Learning Center...(n.d.) Genetically
Modified Food. Retrieved from
http://learn.genetics.utah.edu/content/science/gmfoods/

http://www.gmo-
compass.org/eng/grocery_shopping/fruit_vegetables/14.gen
etically_modified_papayas_virus_resistance.html

Huff. E. (2013) Naturanl News. Retrieved from
http://www.naturalnews.com/040556_arsenic_chicken_fee
d_contamination.html

McClees. H (2015). How to choose a Papaya that's not Genetically Modified. Retrieve from http://www.onegreenplanet.org/vegan-food/how-to-choose-a-papaya-thats-not-genetically-modified/

Mercola. Com (2013). Milk and Dairy Products laced with rBGH. Retrieve from http://articles.mercola.com/sites/articles/archive/2013/07/10/banned-foods.aspx

Natural health website. (2013). Ractopamine: the meat additive banned almost everywhere but America. Retrieve from

http://articles.mercola.com/sites/articles/archive/2013/12/24/ractopamine-beta-agonist-drug.aspx#_edn3

Natural health website. (2013). Salmon Confidential. Retrieve from

http://articles.mercola.com/sites/articles/archive/2013/04/13/salmon-confidential.aspx

Natural health website.(2013). U.S. Foods chockfull of ingredients banned in other countries. Retrieved from http://articles.mercola.com/sites/articles/archive/2013/02/27/us-food-products.aspx

U.S. Agency for Toxic Substances and Diseases Registry (ATSDR). 2005. "Toxicological Profile for Arsenic." http://www.atsdr.cdc.gov/toxprofiles/tp2.pdf.

Wellness. Berkeley. (2011) Two Preservatives to Avoid?. Retrieve from http://www.berkeleywellness.com/healthy-eating/food-safety/article/two-preservatives-avoid

www.ingramcontent.com/pod-product-compliance
Lightning Source LLC
Chambersburg PA
CBHW071323280526
45788CB00004B/2002